Change Your Life With Meditation:

A Step By Step Guide To Calming Your Mind, Reducing Stress, And Living Longer Starting Today!

Jennifer N. Smith

Table of Contents

Introduction

We can all use a little more peace in their lives, and who doesn't want to live longer? There are so many things we all need but are not able to get our hands on, you know? Mostly because these concepts are so insubstantial that it can be difficult for us to accomplish them. Some goals are easy to achieve: saving money by making budget cuts, or losing some weight if we are dedicated to changing our lifestyles. However, these goals will never be able to make us truly happy if we never learn how to be alone with ourselves. Fortunately for us, there is a solution to this problem.

That solution happens to be meditation. The art of meditation has been used for thousands of years as a way to help people get in touch with their spiritual selves, so that they can gain enough insight and peace of mind to move forward in their lives. Meditation has also been used to tackle any problems that they might face. **Without practicing meditation, we might often find ourselves more stressed out than we can deal with, and look for other ways to try and take away the burden of our problems.**

Many people don't like to look inward, and introspection can leave them feeling very unhappy. Of course, we all have certain troubles in our lives; but if we are not able to face them in a healthy way, we will always stay stuck in the same unhappy mindset. If you truly want inner peace, you are going to have to become happy being still within yourself. Otherwise, the rest will be more difficult to accomplish and you will find yourself struggling tremendously along the way. Try not to be discouraged by this, because everybody has a way to make their lives a little bit better. All you have to do is find out for yourself just how to make yourself feel better and change your life. Meditation can help you to do exactly that.

In this book, we will cover everything you need to know about meditation: from how to get into the right mindset so that we can meditate properly, to many of the different techniques that have been utilized over the centuries.

If you are ready to start learning how to utilize meditation for yourself to change your life and find more peace of mind, or you are interested in learning more about the key to living a longer life, then this is the book for you. All you have to do is start today! Once you have understood all of the ways that meditation can benefit you and the changes that you can make, you will be a completely different person. If you allow mediation to become a more integral part of your lifestyle, you will be full of gratitude for the plethora of benefits that this concept can bring into your life.

Meditation Q & A

Q: Can meditation really make us healthier?

A: Yes! You can be definitely sure that practicing meditation can physically benefit our lives.

Q: What is meditation?

A: Simply put, meditation is the art of relaxation and a technique that leaves us receptive to internal wisdom.

Q: Why should I meditate?

A: **Meditation helps us to focus more on the positive and less on the negative!** If we are too focused on the bad - as most of us are - it becomes harder to relieve stress and anxiety. There are also lots of health benefits of meditation that you don't want to miss out on!

Q: What kinds of health benefits are there?

A: Meditation can help us with everything related to our mental, spiritual and physical wellbeing, from improving concentration, relieving stress and anxiety, to extending the length of our lives! Find out more in the book!

Q: How should I look when I'm meditating?

A: Your posture depends on your meditation, as there are many styles to choose from. For the most part, beginners should sit comfortably, usually with their eyes closed. Don't try too hard to hold a position that isn't comfortable. You will get there eventually, but your main focus should be on your comfort level!

Q: How long should I meditate?

A: Meditating is a personal practice that should last as long as you feel comfortable; you should stop when you feel done. Beginners can get their feet wet using short amounts of meditation at first, not more than five minutes long, and work their way up to half an hour, depending on your personal preference!

Q: Do I need a teacher to be an expert meditator?

A: Not at all! Just doing a little research and practicing can set you on the path you need to find better health and enlightenment!

Chapter 1 - Clearing Your Mind

When people think of meditation, I'm pretty sure everyone gets the same mental image on their mind: somebody sitting down in a quiet area with their eyes closed. We all have a very clear idea of what meditation is supposed to look like, and we all know that the first step in achieving a good meditative state is to clear your mind.

There are many reasons that meditation is beneficial to the body, and most of them are physical; some of them also happen to be mental. We spend our days so unnecessarily consumed with the rest of our lives, that we often forget to take the time to stop thinking. In fact, we often forget to simply feel and let go of needless emotions that are just holding us back.

Because of so many consuming emotions inside us, many people don't actually know how to let go of ourselves. It becomes very difficult for us to clear our minds so that we can begin to focus on our inner peace and well-being. Clearing the mind is one of the biggest challenges that most people face when they are trying to learn how to meditate. If you do not know how to clear your mind, meditation may seem just a waste of time. You might as well just be sitting on the couch and watching television rather than sitting down to listen to your own thoughts.

There will still be thoughts passing through our minds when we meditate. We cannot turn your brains off, can we? Clearing our mind is a great goal, but it does take time and practice before we can accomplish this on a whim. **Clearing the mind is one of the hardest elements of meditation for beginners.** We are constantly trying to solve problems in our brains, even when we are busy doing something else. When we are finally allowed to sit down in a quiet space and delve into the mysteries of our minds, a lot of different thoughts and feelings are likely to come into our mind.

The concept of meditation has been known for thousands of years. Even our forefathers from
the hunter-gatherer societies are thought to have benefited from the altered states of consciousness that can be reached through meditation. Of course, clearing the mind is an important first step to reaching these altered states; it should not be overlooked that all of us have a difficult time relaxing directly after a stress-related event.

Think about this for a moment: what part of your day is not stressful? Do you have any moments where you are able to just sit and relax, or is this why you are turning to meditation in the first place? Don't beat yourself up for not being able to relax the second that you close your eyes. Personally, we are constantly stressed out and seeking new ways to relax our bodies and minds; we try to fine-tune our spirits so that we are able to work in direct unity with the goals that are closest to the greater good.

Do you know what's ironic about trying to clear our minds? It's that we generally begin by stressing out about whether or not our mind is clearing fast enough.

Here is the fact: nobody can clear their mind the second they close their eyes unless they have had

many years of experience. When you start to delve deeper into the realms of your psyche, you are going to discover a lot of turbulence along the way. There are thoughts that will show up again and again. We call these circling thoughts. Many times, these circling thoughts are indicators of some patterns that our brain have started to get comfortable with. They are habitual and quite difficult to change over the course of time. Because of this, it is no wonder why they show up when we are trying to clear our minds.

The most important thing for you to do when you are trying to clear your mind is to remember that it will not happen to you immediately. This is completely okay! Do not add more stress to the thoughts in your head. Instead, try one of these techniques to avoid these thoughts and search your mind more deeply.

Exercise Before Meditating

There's something that most people don't think about while meditating. Our bodies will naturally want to relax and seek a meditative state after extreme bouts of exertion. If it is difficult for you to clear your mind, think about how easy it is to keep your mind focused on the task at hand during exercise. Think about how easy it is not to have any thoughts in your mind when you are resting or taking a break while your body recovers from an intense workout. Taking advantage of this for meditation purposes can be very rewarding for a beginner, especially for someone who is searching for ways to help themselves clear their minds.

Try to De-Stress and Relax Throughout the Day

It can be difficult for us to clear our minds if we have had a very stressful day. Fortunately, there are ways that we can do our best to eliminate the stress that we are under, and also try to get rid of the stress we have already encountered. If it is difficult for you to relax throughout the day, it will be more difficult for you to let go and surrender yourself to the powers of meditation. If this is the case, you can try simple things throughout the day that can relax you. Drinking a soothing tea or a glass of warm milk can help, as can taking a short nap. Some people prefer to listen to comforting music, or exercise at home. These will help you at the end of the day when you are finally ready to try some meditation.

Choose the Right Environment

This may sound like obvious thing when you are undergoing a meditation, but choosing the right environment is very important. Sometimes we do not make the right choice right away; often times, we find ourselves in situations that can leave us stressed out with nowhere to turn to. For example, if you have young children in the house and you want to meditate, you might have trouble finding the right time and location. You might have a lot of difficulty sneaking in a short meditation session, particularly if you cannot set aside a soothing environment where you can allow yourself to clear your mind. It is important that you find a location away from distractions and disturbances, even if it is in a park, away from the chaos of home.

The choice is yours, and you can decide for yourself whether or not you want to create an environment close by or choose one that is more relaxing.

Count Your Breaths

One particular method many people try to use to combat insomnia is to focus on your breathing. The reason that breathing helps is that it helps us to go into a slight trance. As we focus our minds more on the hypnotic rhythms of our autonomic body functions, such as breathing, we become completely focused on it. Autonomic body functions, such as blinking and breathing, happen whether we intend for them to or not, as they are vital to our health and well-being. By counting our breaths, we are able to open our minds and focus on the calming state that is produced by the beginning stages of meditation.

Stretch Before Meditation

Before you begin your meditation, you may find it helpful to do a few stretches first. Stretching helps our body to relax and provides us with the ability to unwind. We are also a lot less likely to fidget and feel restless while we are attempting to clear our minds and enter tranquil states of meditation. Stretching can also be useful because it can help us to start focusing on the internal aspects of our bodies rather than staying focused on the external factors.

Sit Somewhere Soft

One of the most important ways to help your mind stay clear when meditating is to rest somewhere soft. If you are sitting on a hard or uncomfortable surface, the physical discomfort can make it even more difficult to clear your mind. Most of us have enough trouble doing this anyway without having to worry about re-adjusting our sitting positions. If you are meditating somewhere comfortable, it will be much easier for you to stay focused.

Understanding these vital ways of clearing our minds can truly help us get where we want to be. Using these tricks, you should be able to find a way to clear your mind quickly and easily. Completely clearing your mind and focusing on your inner thoughts can always be a challenge, even for the most practiced meditator. Understanding these tricks will help us in our journey moving forward on the beginner's path to meditation.

Chapter 2 - Your Meditation Space

It is very important that you have a specific meditation space where you feel safe and comfortable being vulnerable, especially if you don't feel great opening up to yourself and truly exploring your deepest layers. If this is the case, it will be extra difficult for you to be able to clear your mind and get comfortable as you explore the different strategies of meditation. This should never discourage you from trying though, even if you don't think you have a safe and comfortable space. You could always explore the environment around your home and try to find a safe place for yourself.

Your meditation space doesn't have to be a big one. They can actually be very small, so long as it is safe and comfortable. You can meditate in your bedroom or in your bathroom, or even in an office room or at the park. You can use any kind of space to explore your spirituality; however, as it is such a vulnerable and personal process, most people benefit from having a safe space right within their homes. Using a space in your home makes it easily accessible any time and it can physically trigger your body into a state of relaxation when you know it is close to you.

This same concept can be applied to people with insomnia. If you only use your bed for sleeping, it will trigger an automatic and physiological response causing your body to feel sleepy when you are in your bed. People suffering from insomnia are very careful about not using their bed to read, work or watch television. These little habits may seem like nothing from the outside; but from the inside, creating these little areas for ourselves to be safe and comfortable is extremely important.

If you have a separate room that you can use, you can make it fit to your comfort level. You can paint it in your favorite color – something soothing and soft that makes you feel peaceful. You can have speakers in the room that plays soothing music, as well. If you have meditation recordings that you would like to use, this can be extremely beneficial when you are working on your meditation. This is particularly true for beginners, who may not be sure where to begin with their meditations. Make sure to play the music at a gentle volume so that it doesn't actually interrupt your state of tranquility.

In your room, you should also make sure that you have somewhere comfortable to sit. Blankets and pillows can be very useful, because when you are meditating the last thing you want to do is come back unexpectedly into your body because of an ache or pain. You can avoid this by being comfortable.

There is no point in meditating in an uncomfortable space; so, make sure that you have precisely what you need in your meditation space. This will also help you to get into the mindset that you need for your meditation before you ever sit down and get started. Your body will recognize the space and what it is used for and begin to respond accordingly, making your mental work a lot easier.

In your personal meditation space, burning some soothing candles can also be beneficial. Sometimes you can burn incense to help lift you up into the state of tranquility that you are hoping for. Certain smells can be very uplifting during meditation and can help us to reach the altered states of mind that many meditations aim for.

Overall, what's important is that you make your atmosphere soothing and comfortable, and you are able to feel safe there. Even if you need to drape a sheet over a corner for you to have a private corner in your home where you can meditate, you should feel free to do so without any hesitation. What's most vital is that you have a corner or a room where you feel safe and comfortable, and where you can focus on your inner thoughts more than on the outside world.

Meditation is something that can change your life. It not only helps you to find inner peace that we all strive for, but it can also lengthen your lifespan.

Chapter 3 – Soothing Sounds and Music

If you are a beginner and you are finding it difficult to clear your mind, soothing sounds and music can be a great way to help yourself. The right sounds and music can help you to move forward in your meditation journey and get used to the feeling of staying still and vulnerable to yourself. Looking inwardly can be very difficult and exhausting if you are not enjoying yourself, so make sure that you are able to stay relaxed and keep your mind focused when you are meditating.

Because this can be so difficult for beginners, many of the meditation CDs that are out there include music and a soothing voice giving you instructions. These instructions are usually very basic, teaching you to breathe properly and guide your thinking. These instructions are designed to help you to reach a new state of consciousness where you are able to feel yourself as organically as possible. They will help you to distance yourself from any distractions from the outside environment where you usually feel the most stressed out.

Meditation is a way to help you to escape the chaos in your life and to look inwardly so that you can seek solutions and answers to questions you may not even know you have. Each of us suffer at some point in our lives with too much stress and the riddles that life can sometimes throw at us. The tumultuous waves that we ride on every day can be overwhelming without a little bit of help. By using music as a tool to aid us in meditation, we are providing an environment where our brains can stop concentrating on all of the difficulties in our lives, avoid the habitual things that we think about and the compulsive actions we take. **The right music can help us to truly focus inside ourselves on a peaceful well of inspiration and calmness that lies within us at all times, but which we can have trouble finding.**

Most of us lose sight of this aspect of our selves, but it is one of the most beneficial things that the human body is capable of doing. Most beginners do need an aid however, which is where soothing sounds and music can come into play. So if you are interested in music and trying to decide on the type that will help you in your meditations, here are a few examples.

Meditation Recordings

Meditation recordings can help you with your breathing exercises and your focus, as well as guide you on your spiritual journey. There are many different people who have made these recordings, and you can find them very easily. These recordings and tapes can be found in nearly any bookstore or record store in your locality. Most of the time, people who create these tapes are experienced practitioners who want to ensure that you have a successful experience. These are especially beneficial for beginners who have never tried any form of meditation before. If you would like to hear what an experienced person experiences during their meditations, and how they are able to focus enough to reach their state of tranquility, these recordings may be the best for you.

Natural Sounds

Another kind of recording that helps to practice meditation are natural sounds; these kinds of recordings also help people with insomnia or people who can't relax. **The sounds of the earth are tranquil and hypnotic, and can help us to be lulled easily into a state of peacefulness.** Most people have a difficult time reaching this state without help; so, listening to hypnotic, natural noises can truly benefit any beginner at meditation. Try going for things that have a natural rhythm, such as ocean waves and rain drops falling onto a soft surface. These are very steady and calming, and can help you in your meditation.

Music

Certain types of music have also been known as helpful for beginners in meditation to succeed in reaching a tranquil state. Most of these do not include words, but are rather instrumental music that are both relaxing and soothing. They are not songs with a fast tempo, but rather slow and gentle tunes. **The best tracks for meditation are simple and soothing, and they do not have any lyrics.** Sometimes soothing music in a foreign language can put us in a state of tranquility, as we can concentrate on the tune and the music instead of listening to the lyrics.

Now that we have covered the kinds of sounds and music that you can listen to in order to enhance your meditation techniques, you will be more prepared to clear your mind.

Many times, music is a soothing thing, whether we are trying to clear our minds and meditate or for something else. It has been used in many types of therapy as well, and can frequently hold many benefits in our lives. Selecting the right sounds and music to meditate with can help you to reach your state of tranquility as a beginner with ease.

Chapter 4 – Candles

When it comes atmosphere, another very helpful component can be the aid of candles. Candles can change the atmosphere of a room from bleak to comfortable; some candles even come with scents that induce a state of relaxation. Some people use candles during their meditation because they want to encourage a deeper hypnotic trance.

Many people use candles to get rid of any source of artificial lighting and come closer to natural elements. Not only are candles relaxing, but they give both natural light and warmth from live fire. Most people really enjoy candlelight, and find it easy to de-stress when they have candles lit around them. This is also why so many people use candles when taking a relaxing bath or when they are spending a romantic evening with their significant other. There's just something very soothing about candles. **If you want to meditate in a soothing and stress-free environment, sometimes lighting candles is just the way to do that.** It doesn't have to have anything to do with actual candle meditation, although this is also an option.

If you should decide that you would like to use candles for meditation, you may want to take a few things into consideration. Such as, what candle holders do you already have? This will determine the types of candles you should buy. How long would you want to be meditating for and how safe do you feel having candles lit in your meditation space? Do you have a fire alarm or smoke detector in your meditation room? Are there any chemical sensitivities you may have to scented candles? If not, which scents do you prefer? You should always try to go for naturally scented candles rather than the artificially scented candles, because most chemical fragrances are actually toxic. It is best to stay away from chemically enhanced candles at all times; if you do not, it may disrupt your ability to meditate.

There are a lot of options for candles you can have in your meditation space. Some suggestions for relaxing candles would be to light those that smell like lavender. Lavender is a natural aid for stress relief, and when the scent is diffused into the environment, it can create a very relaxing environment. Lavender has been used for many things, including a sleep aid, and this is not surprising. The scent is extremely relaxing and can provide many benefits to the body.

Another aspect to choosing candles can be the color. Many people think that the concept of colors are meaningful in meditation, and our minds associate certain colors with certain feelings. If you are trying to invoke a certain feeling during your meditation sessions, you should try to make sure that you are using the right color. If you have a specific goal, make sure that the color of candle you choose is compatible with the mindset that you hope to invoke.

Some of the generally agreed upon meanings of colours when it comes to choosing a candle are as follows:

- **Blue:** Wisdom and harmony, loyalty, dream realms, healing.

- **Gold:** Money and good luck fast. Business sense. Promotes good understandings.

- **Green:** Fertility, accomplishments, and auspiciousness.

- **Orange:** Balance, success, mental aptitude, and energy or stamina.

- **Pink:** Heartfelt emotions and heightened energy.

- **Purple:** Psychic phenomena, material embodiment of desires. Power.

- **Yellow:** Charm, confidence, attraction, persuasion.

- **Red:** Energy, sensuality, strength, vitality, willpower.

- **White:** Healing and purification. Truth, peace, happiness, and unity.

Chapter 5 – Meditating in the morning

Many people believe that doing some important activity in the morning can help us to harness the vital life energy that can keep us going throughout the day. This is why, different types of **Tai Chi** exercises are usually done in the morning because it is believed that mornings are a special time. **When it comes to meditation, practicing in the morning can actually be a very beneficial process.** If you begin your morning with a clear mind and a sunny disposition, created by a successful meditation of meditation, you are setting yourself up to have a great morning, and potentially a great day. No matter what happens after a good meditation session, it is easier to bounce back.

Sometimes the best practice we can achieve is to learn how to get into a good routine. If we are able to work something new into our morning routine, considering that morning is the time of the day when we have the most routines in place, it is a lot more likely that we will succeed at keeping meditation a part of our daily regimen. **You can even meditate more than once a day, if that is what you prefer.**

Morning meditation can be a great idea, because during this time, you will still be close to a relaxed state. You will easily be able to keep your mind clear and focus on your state of tranquility in the morning. If you choose to meditate in the morning, it is best to do a session that can fill you with energy and give you a positive mindset to face the day with; otherwise. it is possible that you will simply fall right back to sleep! That wouldn't be very helpful for anybody, especially if you have somewhere to be during the rest of your day!

Meditating in the morning is also practical as it is usually the quietest time of the day, where there are generally not as many people rushing around and creating chaos wherever you go. You can take a brisk morning walk to your local park or even practice in your own backyard if you wanted some sunlight. You may find that this is more revitalizing than you ever could have imagined! If this is the case, you will be able to truly appreciate and utilize morning meditation for yourself.

If we are able to meditate in the mornings, it is extra helpful because our minds are not cluttered by the responsibilities we have to take care of throughout the day. We will be able to clear our minds much more easily in the morning. Habits are so easier to form during our morning routines, especially when it is likely for us to become distracted later on in the day. We cannot plan every second of our day; trying to plan our days diligently can be extremely difficult. This can make it very hard for us to integrate a new element to our routine, such as a morning meditation session. However, introducing a morning meditation session in the morning makes it that much easier for you to get settled into a good routine of meditation, especially for beginners. It's the best time to start, for so many amazing reasons!

If you are serious about getting into a good routine and learning more about how morning meditation can work for you, all you have to do is choose the meditation technique that you prefer the most and try it for yourself! You can begin just as soon as you get out of bed. Of course, you can brush your teeth first if you would like to, but meditating first thing in the morning can be extremely helpful for a beginner. It will especially be beneficial for someone who has a difficult time clearing their mind. Everybody has a hard time clearing the mind at some time, but if you want to start getting the full effects of meditation quickly, morning meditation sessions can be the best. It can be one of the fastest ways to finding your inner peace and beginning a routine that can lead you to a longer and healthier life.

Chapter 6 – Gratitude

One of the most important thing that most people won't tell you about meditation is the power of gratitude that comes with it. **Gratitude comes in all shapes and sizes, but when it comes to meditation, we really have a great opportunity to expand our sense of our surroundings. We'll gradually begin to know the way that the world works.** Most of us would do everything possible to make sure that we are able to move forward in our lives with no regrets. We would like to live without any worries and anxieties whatsoever, and have no negativity plague us on a daily basis. That is probably one of the very reasons that you are reading this book. All of us have a hard time dealing with the day-to-day roller coaster ride of human emotion, and we look for a way out of this.

Unfortunately, this is one of the most common aspects of human life. All of us are destined to feel our emotions one way or another – good or bad - and we have no choice but to accept them. If we bury our emotions, we begin to have some issues with ourselves; hiding from our problems eventually turns out to be a lot more trouble than its worth. Dealing with troubling emotions is another time when meditation can become extra beneficial. If you have buried too many deep thoughts and feelings too deeply, meditating can help you to explore these problems in a new light in a safe and comfortable atmosphere. At least in this area, you will be able to begin working on yourself and moving towards solutions to whatever problems may haunting you. It may seem silly, but practicing gratitude can actually help us move forward in this process.

If you have ever gone through a difficult time in your life - just as every one of us has - you will understand that the feelings elicited from those times are usually very difficult to deal with. They may be painful and ugly, just like all negative feelings. The worst part is that we didn't put these feelings there ourselves; most of our sadness seems to be due to situations and circumstances far beyond our control. Even if we had opportunities to make mistakes and feel regret, these things can plague us and cause us to feel a great amount of grief. This is where gratitude really comes in handy.

It may seem silly to believe that everything happens for a reason, or that there is still anything good to think about left in this world. We may encounter many problems along the way as we try to unpack the issues that our pain has caused us. However, if we are able to practice mindfulness and cultivate a sense of gratitude for all of the blessings we still have, the negative events will not seem so bad anymore. It may seem way too simple to work, and yet it is exactly what happens. People who meditate and think about gratitude are more likely to be able to move on after difficult events, and even find a sense of peace and happiness. This inner peace can provide us with a longer life and the ability to move confidently into new situations rather than being afraid of them.

Most people are terrified of making the same mistakes over and over again. However, the only way we learn how to live is through our own mistakes and experiences. Without these to fall back on, we become dangerous and vulnerable to a world that may continue to hurt us. Unfortunately, living this way actually decreases our happiness; it also makes it a lot more difficult for us to tap into the vulnerability that makes our life beautiful. This vulnerability is what we need in order to stay happy in a world that is full of problems. If we were able to be honest about how we feel and express ourselves easily and honestly, many of the issues in our lives would simply disappear. If we are too afraid to allow ourselves to be vulnerable and trusting, we are setting ourselves up for more problems further on down the line.

Practicing gratitude can help us to remember that there are many things in our lives that have gone right. Most of us become fixated on the bad, to the point that we glaze over the good things; we only remember the hard times that we have experienced, not the good. We don't believe that things will ever be right again, just because we have had the carpet pulled out from under us. It's difficult to be left on the ground, stunned and confused about why we are suffering. None of us ever expect the worst to happen. When it does, it can be very difficult to reconcile with it. We may become obsessed with the bad things that have happened to us, re-create old pains over and over again, because of our unwillingness or inability to process and heal from them.

By practicing gratitude, and allow yourself to meditate on the things in our lives that are worth celebrating, we are opening ourselves up. We are actually allowing more good into our lives. If you want to meditate and change your life, you will have to accept that there are probably things that you are holding on to that you don't need. These things can be damaging and hold you back from new experiences. On the other hand, there are types of vulnerability that can leave you happy and content in a way you may never have thought possible.

Gratitude is celebrated in most major religions, and there is a good reason for this. If we are able to feel grateful for what we have, we will no longer feel pained about the things we do not have, or everything that have gone wrong. When we really count them, our blessings far outweigh our failures. **Remembering this can give us a renewed faith that there is good in the world; with that thought in our mind, we will finally be able to move forward in our life and continue to reap blessings everywhere we go.** The world is full of miracles and gifts, but without gratitude it is difficult for us to understand and believe this. We go into a deep and dark place far within our own minds which is difficult to come out from. However, meditating on gratitude can help us to break out of this dark place and appreciate all the great things about our lives. Unnecessary

It can be one of the most important aspects of changing our lives and living a healthier life than our peers. It's a huge shift in perspective that can bring us more joy and abundance than anything else that we could do for ourselves. Most of us have a difficult time believing that the world is actually working in our favor; in fact, most of us are certain that it is working against us. However, if you think about it, if you are actually getting yourself up from off the ground, and pulling yourself up by the bootstraps the old-fashioned way, you will be able to seek many opportunities with a clear mind. **We have the power to turn things around, and instead of letting things happen to us, we can begin to make them happen *for* ourselves!**

Not being able to feel or show gratitude can cause a lot of problems in your life. It can cause you to isolate yourself from friends and loved ones, feeling as if you may not be receiving as much as you should be. But before you think about this, maybe you should consider another fact: is it possible that you are not giving as much as you have received? How much do you give that makes you eligible to receive so much?

Gratitude and generosity are closely tied. The world is actually very generous to each and every one of us only if we are perceptive enough to the gifts we get. Whether you believe there is something in the universe working in our favor or not, the balance of the world is undeniable. Balance is a scientific concept that governs our world and lives. Without acknowledgment of the good and overindulgence of the bad, we may find ourselves suffering needlessly. These sufferings can be easily avoided if we were just able to understand and practice gratitude more frequently in our daily lives.

Practicing gratitude can also be tied with mindfulness. Every day, you could try and pick out all of the things that have made you happy or that you have noticed that are beautiful. You could think about all of the things that other people have done to make you smile or all the support you have received from loved ones. Instead of thinking about how difficult it is for you to connect with people, maybe you can try and make a new connection and feel all of joys and benefits of a new social interaction with someone new.

Even if it doesn't work out the way you wanted it to, you can be grateful that you have a living body that you can use to navigate the world. Try and be grateful for all of the things that you have received from the world instead of being resentful for the things that you want and have not acquired yet.

It will change your life forever, and help you to live a longer, healthier and more rewarding life.

Chapter 7 – Wandering Thoughts

If you are new to meditation, the idea of having to clear your mind may seem distressful. You may feel very inadequate or unhappy with yourself for not being able to clear your mind right away. We tried to shed some light on the stigma of clearing the mind in the first chapter, but for the most part, none of us will be able to clear our minds right away. This is absolutely normal, and actually the sign of a healthy brain. All of us have wandering thoughts, and they wander wherever they want to and however they want to. This happens to us when we are in class and should be paying attention, or when we are talking to somebody but our attention drifts from the conversation. So, it is no different when this happens during meditation!

The first trick to dealing with wandering thoughts is to stop making such a big deal out of them. Everybody has wandering thoughts, and none of us will be able to clear our minds immediately, especially if we are a beginner. No matter who we are, you can always have a random thought popping into your head, no matter how still and quiet our mind seems to be. We are always perceiving the things that are happening around us, consciously or otherwise. All of us are able to pick up on signals from our environment that may or may not trigger a neural response to those events. Each of us has a new opportunity every moment to observe or listen to, or pick up some kind of activity around us. Therefore, it is not very surprising that clearing our mind is almost impossible.

When we are practicing mindfulness meditation in particular, wandering thoughts are free to come and go as they please. We should stop making such a big deal out of random thoughts, and stop stressing out about the fact that they exist. **Nobody is able to fully control the way they think all the time.** This can happen for many different reasons, and all of us have our own biases and prejudices that were planted there by other people from when we were young. This doesn't mean that we are inherently flawed; no matter how we are raised, we are still going to function in our lives as unique individuals. The issue with this is that sometimes these thoughts and processes are unwanted, but we still have to live with them.

If you do discover yourself having unwanted thoughts every time you want to meditate, and you would like to get rid of them, meditation may actually be a great way to help you address this problem. If these thoughts refuse to leave your mind when you are meditating, you will probably be able to find them inside your head. You will be able to follow them somewhere deep inside yourself, from the origin of where that thought came from and why you might think that way. The thought might negatively impact your life, but it will not leave you easily. If you want to change this, you can do so; it's not easy, but it is possible. Meditation can help you to understand the root of your issues and follow through with an effective solution.

If you allow yourself to listen to your wandering thoughts, you will be able to have a more peaceful mind and a less wavering focus on the meditation at hand. Wandering thoughts are absolutely normal and should not make you angry just because they are there. Instead, you should just listen to what your body is saying, because this is often something that you need to pay attention to. Everybody has some kind of random train of thought in their mind that is always going on; if you want to start changing the way that your wandering thoughts interfere with your life because they are not being helpful, you will be able to recognize the wandering or invasive thought during your everyday routine and replace it with a different and more positive thought.

Doing this can change the neural pathways in your brain so that you do not continue to suffer from the same circling thoughts over and over again. This can help you to cut back a lot of the anxiety that you feel during your daily life; without so many random thoughts bothering you, you can move forward in a more peaceful way than you ever thought possible before. Most of us have a difficult time understanding our limitations and the ways that our brain sometimes works against us out of habit. Even if you feel like the universe is working against you, the chances are more likely that you are working against yourself. Many of us sabotage ourselves without even realizing it, and addressing and paying attention to our wandering thoughts during meditation can help us to shed some light into the reasons why and the ways that we are limiting ourselves.

Meditation can also help us have a stronger connection to the positive sides of our life. If we are able to recognize that a majority of our thoughts are negative, and we can intercept them throughout the day with more positive ideas, there is nothing to stop us from becoming the best form of ourselves that we can possibly be. All in all, meditation helps us to reduce stress and keep a healthier and happier outlook on life, even on the day-to-day basis, without doing all the difficult work of deconstructing our wandering thoughts.

Just allowing ourselves time to sit down and process some of our emotions is highly beneficial. Most of us don't give ourselves enough time to do this in an adequate way. This leaves us muddled and full of excess energy that gets expelled in the wrong ways. This can sometimes lead to difficulties in our relationships and our surroundings. If we are not happy inside, then we are not happy outside; It is more difficult for us to make the healthy connections that we need in order to grow.

Overall, wandering thoughts are not something that you should be stressed out about. This can seriously endanger your ability to let go and reach an altered state of consciousness through meditation. **You should always just acknowledge the fact that you have had a thought and let it pass undisturbed,** unless you want to use your meditation as an opportunity to follow that thought. You can use mindfulness meditation to find out where that thought leads you to discover more about yourself than you might have known originally. All of us have a difficult time at some point in our lives, and if we are able to really examine this, meditation can truly take a huge weight off our shoulders. Reflecting inwardly can encourage a deeper form of inner peace than we might have known was possible before we began our meditation.

Chapter 8 – The Benefits of Meditation: Relieving Anxiety, Stress, and More

If you are a beginner to meditation, you may understand that anxiety and stress can be reduced through meditation. Yes, this seems to be very intuitive and easy to understand, but there is actually a particular field of science that can back up this fact. Meditation can help us soothe our anxiety, relieve ourselves from stress, and have a whole lot of amazing health benefits. **If you have ever wondered why this is, in a more scientific aspect, then this is the chapter that will explain how meditation can physiologically and psychologically change our lives.**

When we meditate, a lot of the time we are faced with the wandering thoughts mentioned in the previous chapters. When we are able to address these thoughts and allow them to pass through us, it allows us a certain amount of freedom that we never had before. Accepting and acknowledging our thoughts and allowing them to continue on their way without troubling ourselves over them can be an extremely crucial exercise in relieving stress and anxiety.

Most sources of stress and anxiety come from fear. We are either afraid of the future or afraid of what may happen to us as a direct result of our past. Often times, we have a difficult time with stress and anxiety and it can manifest into physical symptoms that can shorten our lifespan; stress can actually make us numb to the outside world. Most of us are always constantly looking for a way to address our fears so that we can have a happier and more fulfilling life. Even if we do not realize the fears that we harbor, they are without a doubt constantly plaguing us and affecting the way that we live our lives.

If we were able to live without these fears and anxieties, we would be able to follow a path of mindfulness that would provide us with a great sense of well-being and security. People with anxiety severely lack a sense of security. **Security is difficult for people with anxiety to attain because they are so lost in their own thoughts; these people are not paying attention to the present moment**. When we don't know how to pay attention to the present, we become overwhelmed by the tides of the past or the worry for the future.

Although it can be a good thing for us to start to deconstruct our past and live a happier and healthier life, doing so becomes a lot easier with time. We don't always understand the way our anxiety is affecting us, so it can also be beneficial to have some help from somebody who can bounce ideas off you. Someone experienced can help you understand your perspective in a new light. Maybe there are flaws in your thinking that you didn't realize you had and you wanted to address them to become happier. It would be difficult to do so without some feedback, for which you need the help of someone experienced in meditation and mindfulness. Without meditation, you may not realize there are any problems at all. That would make it impossible for you to improve and find yourself in a happier position in life. A lot of people don't know the source of their real troubles, and they blame all the wrong things in their life for their misery. They never turn their eyes inwardly to understand how they themselves might be negatively impacting the situations that they find themselves in.

Meditation gives us the opportunity to look inside us without having to feel silly or weird about sharing emotions with other people. It gives us a safe and quiet space to begin to process our lives and our experiences. Even if we are going into meditation with an interior goal in mind, such as training ourselves to become adept at perceiving an altered state of consciousness, we are still going to have to do so through a deep inner journey that nobody else can have a say in. We are ultimately going to become the masters of our own domains and our own minds, and meditation is one of the most powerful ways to empower us. It can help us make the decisions that are right for us to move forward in a happier and healthier lifestyle.

Once we are able to start making better decisions, it will reduce the stress that we feel exponentially. The stress that we feel will no longer have control over us and we will feel more empowered in our own lives. When we feel empowered and in control, the symptoms of anxiety also seemed to vanish magically. Our ability to stay in control of our minds and continue to stay in the present and the here and now, can allow us to truly address the anxiety that has before kept us in chains. Meditation can allow us to look at our lives and our experiences in a completely new light so that we can move forward without worry about what might happen in the future. We won't have to worry about that, because our focus is on the "present".

Physically, meditation can also benefit us by decreasing blood pressure and helping us to slow our respiratory rate - which can be a great help in reducing stress and the effects of other disorders. Your blood cortisol levels will also decrease, and your blood circulation will improve as a result of all of these things. If you have a tendency to sweat a lot or if you suffer from an irregular or quickened heartbeat, meditation can even lower your heart rate and promote a deeper state of relaxation to go along with it.

Meditation has also been noted to improve the immune system in general, which is what we use to fight off various disorders and diseases. It is unclear why it has this incredible benefit, but overall meditation helps our bodies and minds to fight off diseases and keep us healthier for longer. All of us are able to reap the rewards of meditation as they carry us away from the dangers of being vulnerable to diseases, helping us to stay healthier overall and avoiding the same complications that can shorten other people's lifespans.

Meditating has also been linked to a more impressive ability to concentrate. It helps us to fine-tune our minds so that we can focus more directly on the tasks at hand and complete them without distractions. Concentration is particularly useful to people who are constantly trying to improve themselves and get through a grueling day at work or school. Without concentration on our side, we often lose sight of the projects that are the most meaningful to us and become overall very unhappy with ourselves and our lives. This type of unhappiness can result in stress and anxiety, which can physically harm the body. Meditation can help to prevent that!

Most illnesses are exacerbated by stress and anxiety, and so it is silly to think that meditation cannot help you. If you are able to improve your state of mind to combat any illness that you face, and to concentrate on the positive rather than the negative, you can see significant improvements to any illnesses and your overall health very quickly in most cases. The power of positive thinking should never be overlooked, and the act of meditation can help us to enhance our powers of positive concentration and allow us to focus on solutions; it can help us to stay dedicated to a healthier and more rewarding lifestyle.

Sometimes, we even add suffering onto the problems we face that does not need to be there. This can impact us deeply and cause us a lot of troubles that speeds up the progression of illness. Meditating helps us in every aspect of disease fighting and prevention, and gives us more benefits that we can even imagine. If we are dwelling on something that makes us unhealthier, meditation can help us to address and avoid this.

With these issues being addressed through meditation, we will be able to truly seek and discover happiness in places that we might have thought were barren in our lives. By applying the concepts of mindfulness and gratitude, stress and anxiety can become a thing of the past.

The techniques in the next section will allow you to utilize these ideas in your meditation practices so that you, as a beginner, can start to reap all the benefits of meditation for yourself. Meditation only gets better with time; stress and anxiety can also become easier with time, and become easier to combat and manage, and ultimately avoid.

Chapter 9 – Dedicating Yourself to Your Meditation Practice

If you are just a beginner to meditation, many of these concepts and ideas may seem novel. You may want to dabble in them until you feel comfortable, and that is perfectly fine. Most of us have a hard time accepting new things as truth and integrating them into our daily rituals and habits. It can take up to two weeks to start a new habit, and staying dedicated to meditation may take even longer than that, especially if you are particularly discouraged by your inability to focus on clearing your mind and allowing your wandering thoughts to come and pass as if they are just the most natural thing in the world. Staying in the present moment and practicing mindfulness every day can seem like an exhausting way to live your life, until you actually learn how to do it and it becomes a second nature to you. Without mindfulness, we have a lot more opportunities to become lost inside ourselves, both in the pain of the past or the fear of the future.

None of us deserve to be lost in the tidal waves of emotions that come with the baggage of the past or the fear and anxiety we feel when facing an uncertain future. These are the most stressful situations that we put ourselves in, and yet this is a habit that most of us have fallen into over the years. We have no control over the past or the future, at least not always. Some things may not happen for us that might be out of our control. Things might not happen for us because we have not taken the time to train yourselves to believe that because anything is possible, it might as well be the thing that we want to happen. It can be very difficult for us to be self-starters, because not everyone has the dedication to something long enough to see it reach fruition. Meditation can help us to change that.

Staying dedicated to a meditation practice can help us to become stronger and wiser, and more capable of taking the challenges in our life head-on so that we can move forward and make a real difference in our lives. If we are unable to stay dedicated to meditation practice, it will be easy for us to fall back into old habits and lose ourselves along the way. None of us want to be unhappy with the way that we live our lives, and sometimes the only thing that we can do to change how we feel about our world is to change the circumstances in which we live. Through meditation, we will be able to really allow ourselves the time to process our lives and understand the source of the anxieties and stresses that we deal with on a day-to-day basis. Meditation can also provide us with much needed time away from these problems and allow us to feel calmer and less stressed out about the problems that we face. It will give us a clear direction to go in, and that direction is toward peace.

If we are constantly moving toward peace and working toward a better state of mind, our bodies can naturally sense this and we feel better than we have in months, or even years. If we are able to bring ourselves peace and joy, then we are no longer feeling powerless in our own lives. However, we have to stay dedicated to the practices that work for us. Sometimes we start to feel discouraged and we simply walk away, or we skip the whole thing, ultimately leading us to giving up a meditation for months or even years. This can be very dangerous, and it is a cycle that we should break as quickly as possible. We do not want to be endangered by our own vicious cycles and habits. If we do not train ourselves to meditate regularly, then it is likely that we will begin to feel overwhelmed even more frequently than is necessary.

To keep meditation a top priority and a habit, you can create a bulletin board that can give you encouragement and remind you why it is important to stay on a path of well-being.

All of us deserve a happy and a healthy life. If you have a hard time staying dedicated to things, you can try a new attempt at committing yourself to meditation. You can put the days that you want to meditate on your calendar. You could set an alarm for the times when you are supposed to stop and drop everything so that you can have some moments of peace. You can write it on a Post-it note and put it on your bathroom mirror so that you remember that you are worth the benefits of meditation. You can have friends and family members ask you how your meditation is going so that you are held accountable to staying dedicated to a routine that will change your life. You can put notes on your bulletin board that encourage you to stay in a positive mindset to practice meditation so that you do not get overwhelmed by the realities of human life. There are a lot of ways to make meditation a part of your life if you want to.

First and foremost, you have to be able to be willing to set time aside and just do it. Even if you don't feel like it, just start. Of course, meditation is the most beneficial if you are able to really jump into it with enthusiasm. But all the stress and anxiety isn't going to go away on its own if you do not stay dedicated to the practice of removing it from your life. Setting time aside to feel tranquil and happy, and to remind yourself that every moment can be a moment of pure joy and happiness is a lot more important than you might think. Not only will it help your mental state of mind, but it will also improve your health and encourage you to change your lifestyle to one that is so healthy that it will add years onto your life. That is something we all deserve, whether we think so or not, so take care of yourself and dedicate yourself to a meditation practice today.

Chapter 10 – Zen Meditation

When we begin to talk about meditation, most of us think of the word "Zen." This is because Zen meditation has been used for thousands of years. Everybody who have practiced Zen has found that it produces amazing results, especially if your hope is to find harmony and balance. Zen is a concept that all of us are familiar with in some way or another, and the purpose of Zen in our lives is to provide us with intrinsic balance and harmony that may otherwise escape us. Even if we do not fully understand the depth of the Eastern philosophies, the take away most of us have is that having Zen in our lives is good.

Simplified, Zen is considered a form of balance. It is similar to the concept of "Yin and Yang", who are able to complement each other in a way that promotes balance and unity even among opposites. It is the concept of chaos being brought to harmony, and every action having an equal and opposite reaction. **Every up has a down, and every left has a right.** By focusing on the balance in the world, we are able to open our minds to some of the most divine concepts of paradox that there are. None of us will ever fully understand or appreciate the way the universe works, because none of us were the ones who created it. The best we can do is try and figure it out for ourselves. The one real concept that has not been disputed over millions of years is that balance plays a key role in the way we live our lives. If we are not balanced, we become unhappy.

Most of us have an intuitive grasp on this idea. We know that if we are never sad, we will never fully appreciate our happiness. We know that without counting our blessings, our curses will pile up and the imbalance can ultimately destroy our lives. The concept of Zen meditation is an important one because this inner awareness within us all is very difficult to reach during the day-to-day lifestyle most of us are busy living. It is too full of stress and action. Most of us do not take the time to sit down and feel aware of every emotion and thought that trickles through our minds. What many of us don't realize is that there is more going on than just what we are able to acknowledge on a normal basis. Unfortunately, our physiological bodies are not all there is to it. We also have a spiritual and inner self that needs attention whether we realize it or not.

This is where Zen meditation comes in handy. By practicing Zen meditation and allowing ourselves to clear our minds and focus inwardly, our spiritual selves will finally have a chance to show up and tell us exactly what we need in order to improve our lives. There is a deep well of wisdom and insight deep within us all, and if we are too busy to stay connected to that well, then we become distracted and unable to progress in our lives. Most of us will stay stuck in an unhappy situation, leaving us disconnected from the most important things that we can do to heal ourselves.

Using Zen meditation, we will be able to tap into the deepest spiritual selves and our bodies. This plethora of unending wisdom within us all becomes easier and easier to access during our daily lives. That is why Zen meditation is one of the most popular types of meditation, both in the Western and Eastern world combined. Everybody needs to be more in touch with their balanced and Zen side, and if you are not able to quickly and easily get in touch with that aspect of yourself, then it is a lot harder for you to make good decisions on a whim. However, if you are able to access your insight into the greater good, it will help you to navigate your life with a lot fewer problems along the way.

Practicing Zen meditation is easy. Here are the steps to follow for a successful Zen meditation practice:

1. Sit somewhere comfortable, such as on a pillow or a cushion that will help you to stay in a meditative state for as long as possible.

2. Choose your favorite meditation posture. One of the most preferred postures for this meditation is the lotus position, which also happens to be the most comfortable position.

3. Rest your hands in a circle in front of your abdomen. This is known as the cosmic mudra. It will help you to receive vital life energy that is full of universal wisdom.

4. Study your breathing and begin to clear the thoughts away from your mind. It can be particularly helpful if you count your breathing. Choose a number to end back before cycling back to one, in case clearing your mind is too difficult. This will allow you to continue the practice and create a steady rhythm that will help you to stay relaxed and peaceful.

5. Once you are able to do this naturally, allow yourself to breathe in and out slowly, focusing simply on the feeling of being still. That is how you do a successful Zen meditation.

Chapter 11 – Mindfulness and Mindfulness Meditation

Have you ever been walking down the street or doing something active and then suddenly had a very powerful sense of where you were right that moment on earth? Maybe you realized that the trees were blowing a certain way and that you are standing in a moment that will never be again. Possibly you were standing with a loved one and just cherishing the present moment and enjoying the smell of their body or the way that the sun was lighting up their hair at just that moment. **These moments are small glimpses into mindfulness. They are what make every day and every new moment a joy and an adventure.**

A simple definition of mindfulness is the ability to experience the present moment as fully as possible. Mindfulness meditations allow us to become immersed in the presence and the beauty of the here and now. This is something that can help many people, especially those who have gone through trauma or other difficult experiences. It is particularly helpful because these people more than anybody need the opportunity to experience life without any baggage of the past weighing them down. If you are able to move forward freely, the painful feelings you experience when you recollect the past can completely disappear.

If we are able to learn how to be completely mindful, our perspectives will become even more objective and we will be able to experience our lives in a whole new way. It can be difficult for many people to experience mindfulness as a way of life. Most of us go on autopilot throughout the day and do our best not to worry about the next step. This is great in the sense that it can protect us from painful thoughts and feelings, but this defense mechanism can actually be dangerous and inhibit our way of life. **If you are able to experience mindfulness, this means that you are able to truly cherish and turn every moment of your life around toward the positive.**

Sadness is sometimes a choice that we make, and it's one that we don't need to make as often as we do. If we live our lives mindfully, we will realize that in any small segments of time, there is no real reason to feel pain or sadness. Without our lives weighed down by pain and sadness, there is a whole lot more time for us to be happy and focus on the aspects of our lives that truly matter. In this aspect, mindfulness can truly change our lives.

When we are NOT living in the present, everything in our lives can be affected. We do not always pay much attention to other people and the way that we affect them, and we are not able to fully process the ways that we are affected by our surroundings. **If we can take each moment bit by bit, one step at a time, and we would chew and swallow it right away instead of letting it build up into a big mass that we choke on, our lives take on a completely new feeling.**

We are so much more open to happiness and positivity, and we are able to feel grateful for the gifts that we receive in every moment. If you sit in a room during an emotional storm, and you take the time to just sit and feel yourself and your body being present in that moment, you will realize that there is nothing truly there to make you unhappy. **Nothing**

is happening to you at that moment. You probably have everything that you need, and the future is in the future and the past is in the past. In the present moment, all you can really know is that you are alive and you are breathing; that in itself is a gift.

Mindfulness meditation will help us to live our lives to the fullest so that we can make the best decisions for ourselves possible. It's very difficult for us to be happy if we are not living the way that we want to live. Living in fear is the fastest way for us to be unhappy, and we will make terrible decisions because either we feel we are not worth the hope of a positive future, or we feel we deserve negativity because of a bad past. If it's time for us to get rid of the chains that keep us in terrible habits and mental patterns, mindfulness meditation is the way to do that.

Here are the steps for a successful mindfulness meditation:

1. Seek out a calm meditation space where you will enjoy exploring your mindfulness meditation. Make sure that it is comfortable and you are seated somewhere that will not harm your body over time if you are unable to move. Also make sure that you won't be disturbed or distracted by anyone else in the process.

2. Choose a position that is comfortable for you - one that is relaxed but upright.

3. Rest your hands somewhere comfortable, preferably on your lap. Make sure that the palms are facing down rather than up. This is the universal position of meditating.

4. Allow your eyes to wander the room, resting wherever they want to rest without thinking too much about whatever it is that you're looking at. It is okay for your eyes to wander.

5. If you begin to lose focus, gently remind yourself that you are attempting mindfulness meditation. The thoughts that you have should be allowed to come and pass as natural, without you adding any input to them whatsoever. Do not follow where these thoughts lead, just let them come and go. Don't pressurize your mind for anything.

6. Focus your attention on to your physiological responses. Think about your breath and how it feels, and think about your heart beat and how steady it is within your body. Allow yourself to truly feel everything in the moment just as it is, and allow yourself to let go of any reluctance you have to do so and believe that everything is all right just how it is.

7. If you begin to get distracted by your thoughts, focus again on your breath and your physiological responses to the meditation. This will help you to stay calm and focused, and help to keep you practiced at staying present in the moment rather than being drawn inwardly to old habits that need broken. Begin practicing if you want to move forward with a more peaceful state of mind.

Chapter 12 – Loving-kindness Meditation

In the previous section, we talked a lot about gratitude. Gratitude is one of the most important aspects of Loving-Kindness meditation. It helps us to open our hearts and minds to loving and accepting all things in creation. Everything that is alive deserves to be loved, and focusing on Loving-Kindness meditation can help us to soften our hard edges. This way, we can begin to accept and acknowledge the fact that love and kindness have a huge place in the world around us. Without it, we stay stuck in terrible traps that prevent us from reaching out to the people around us and create many issues with the world and society at large.

Most Buddhist monks are vegetarian, and Loving-kindness meditations are a way that they continue to maintain the philosophy that everything that is alive is full of love and worthy of love. They believe that everything that is alive presents the world with tremendous gifts and balance that we should always appreciate and cherish. Most of us have a difficult time being vulnerable in the world, as we mentioned before. It can cause a lot of problems and make our lives a lot more difficult to lead comfortably. It is the belief of many that life was formed through love, from the ultimate good, the source of all divinity and kindness. It is only a rift from this source of love and positivity that creates darkness within us that can seem impossible to overcome.

Most of this darkness is due to pain that we do not know how to heal; it may be because it is too difficult for us to feel vulnerable about these problems. If we were truly able to humble ourselves and move forward in a path of healing, Loving-kindness meditation could bring us to the next step in our evolution as an important species. Generosity and an open heart can provide us with the same love and comfort that we have come to cherish from other people. If we are able to give to others, receiving in return takes on a whole new meaning. We understand what it truly means to give and we do not take advantage of the people who have gone out of their ways to provide for us.

Loving-kindness is a way for us to humble ourselves to the helpless. Every single one of us has been helpless at some time in our lives, and if we are unable to provide the same protection and nourishment that we were provided with during our helpless times, it can create a disunity within the world that is difficult to reconcile. All of us deserve to have our needs met, and nobody should be forced to accept less than they deserve because some people want to take more. By practicing Loving-kindness meditation, each of us is able to truly open our minds and hearts to concepts that can bring our world closer toward peace and further away from the disjointed darkness that happens when we are disconnected from our hearts and our divine source of love. Believing such a simple concept can actually make us feel happier on the inside – that has been proven before.

To stay close to our well of Loving-kindness so that we can present the best face possible to the world to the people who deserve the best of us, **Loving-kindness meditation can help us by providing an instant connection to our compassionate natures.** It is natural for us to be compassionate and supportive. Human beings did not develop and evolve with ideas to harm others so that we can progress as a species. Instead, we had to rely on cooperation and teamwork as a species to survive to the point where we are today. If we take advantage of this, we are ignoring Loving-kindness and gratitude and disrespecting the thoughts of our ancestors. Every single one of us should make a more active effort to practice Loving-kindness, so that we can move forward in our evolution and begin to understand how our actions truly affect the rest of the world.

Loving-kindness meditation can be achieved using these simple steps:

1. Go to your meditation space and make sure that you are comfortable. If you would like to light a candle or play some music, you may do so.

2. Take a few deep breaths, slowly and deeply, exhaling until your entire breath is out of your body. Once you feel calm and relaxed, close your eyes.

3. In your heart, think of things that have made you feel loving and grateful. These things can include anything from random acts of kindness, to loving words or compliments that you have received from other people. You can think of the generous love that you have probably received from animals and children all around you. This pure type of love is the key to understanding Loving-kindness meditation. Love given to others without having received first is something to truly be cherished.

4. Hold onto the feeling that these acts bring into your

awareness. Make a vow to return the same type of love into the world, and make this promise at least three times before you take another deep breath and your meditation. It can help you to devote yourself to acting out Loving-kindness in your daily life; and practicing mindfulness as you go throughout your day can help you to understand when Loving-kindness is the best option for you to take.

Conclusion

Every beginner should know all of these amazing techniques of meditation, and especially how they can influence our lives. It can be very difficult to navigate the world when we are full of stress and negative emotions which we don't know what to do with. Fortunately, meditation provides a great escape for us so that we can both get away from the stress of our daily lives and start working on the issues within us.

Allowing ourselves to benefit from the gifts that meditation can bring to our lives is not only good for us; it is also good for the rest of the world. One kind act can have a ripple effect, creating the desire in other people to pass the act forward and provide more joy and generosity into the world. Without these simple acts, many people find it difficult to remember that the world can be a fun and a positive place to live in, full of love, happiness and beauty. This can make the world extra stressful, which can have a direct result on everybody around you. Try not to let yourself fall into this trap. Spread Loving-kindness and Gratitude today!

By meditating, you will not only begin to improve your peace of mind and lower the dangerous possibilities of complications due to stress and anxiety, but you will also begin to start spreading the message that the world very deeply needs to hear. All of us need reminded that there is beauty and love out in the world waiting for us, if only we know where to look.

Meditating can help you to provide opportunities to both yourself and other people to improve your lives and learn how to enjoy the world we live in today!